ANITA MARK

HEALING NATURALLY WITH ACUPRESSURE MADE SIMPLE FOR BEGINNERS

A Guide to Self-Care Ailments

This book is dedicated to anyone on a quest for better health, inner balance, and well-being. May the knowledge within these pages serve as a guiding light on your journey to understanding, practicing, and benefiting from the ancient wisdom of Acupressure. May you find relief, relaxation, and transformation in the gentle touch of your own hands, and may this knowledge bring harmony to your body, mind, and spirit.

Dedicated with warmth and appreciation to all who seek to heal from acupressure

Contents

Acknowledgement

I extend my heartfelt gratitude to all those who contributed to the creation of this book on Acupressure. This journey would not have been possible without the support, guidance, and inspiration from many individuals. My appreciation goes to:

My family and friends for their unwavering encouragement and understanding throughout this endeavor.

The dedicated practitioners and experts in the field of Acupressure who generously shared their knowledge and experiences.

The readers and learners who have shown interest in the healing art of Acupressure, spurring me to share this valuable information.

1

Chapter 1

Introduction

Amidst the bustling streets of a modern metropolis, there exists a timeless practice that transcends the boundaries of science and art, weaving a tapestry of healing and balance. It's not a legend or a secret whispered in hushed tones; it's a remarkable journey into the depths of human connection with the body's own wisdom.

Imagine a young woman named Maya, entangled in the relentless dance of life's demands. Day in and day out, her shoulders bore the weight of deadlines and expectations, her mind a storm of worries and fears. She was adrift in the chaos of the 21st century, seeking refuge from the tempest that raged within her.

One fateful day, Maya stumbled upon a hidden gem, not in a distant land, but within the very core of her existence. Acupressure, an ancient art of healing, beckoned to her like a whispered promise of tranquility. Without knowing it, she embarked on a journey that would forever change her perception of self-care and well-being.

Acupressure, often considered the gentle cousin of acupuncture, proved to be an exquisite portal to a world where touch held the power to unlock vitality, reduce pain, and cradle the spirit. Its secrets were woven into a symphony of pressure points, meridians, and techniques as diverse as the colors of a sunrise.

This is not just a story; it's an invitation to explore a world where the gentle caress of fingertips can silence the cacophony of stress, where the body's wisdom becomes a map to tranquility, and where Maya's journey mirrors your own. Welcome to the captivating realm of acupressure, where the threads of the ancient meet the canvas of the present to paint a picture of well-being, one touch at a time.

What is Acupressure

Acupressure is a holistic healing technique that originates from traditional Chinese medicine. It involves applying manual pressure to specific points on the body, known as acupressure points or pressure points. These points are believed to be connected to pathways of energy, called meridians, which flow throughout the body.

The primary goal of acupressure is to promote wellness and alleviate various health issues by restoring the balance of energy within the body. By applying pressure to these specific points, acupressure is thought to stimulate the body's natural healing mechanisms, relieve pain, reduce tension, and improve overall well-being.

Acupressure does not involve the use of needles, unlike acupuncture, which is a related practice. Instead, it relies on the practitioner's fingers, palms, elbows, or special tools to exert pressure on the identified points. This practice is non-invasive and is often used for a wide range of conditions, including stress, headaches, pain management, and promoting relaxation.

While acupressure is based on ancient Chinese traditions, it has gained recognition and popularity in various parts of the world as a complementary and alternative therapy. It's valued for its natural approach to healing and its potential to help individuals find relief from various physical and emotional ailments.

The History of Acupressure

The history of acupressure is a fascinating journey through the annals of traditional Chinese medicine, dating back thousands of years. Its roots can be traced to ancient China, where it was developed as a holistic healing practice deeply intertwined with the principles of energy balance and meridian systems.

1. Ancient Origins: Acupressure, along with acupuncture, originated in China during the Neolithic period. The earliest records of this practice can be found in texts such as the "Huangdi Neijing" (Yellow Emperor's Classic of Internal Medicine), which dates back to around 200 BCE. This ancient text describes the concept of vital energy, or "qi," and the use of acupressure points to regulate it.

2. Meridian System: Acupressure is built upon the belief in a network of energy channels or meridians that run throughout the body. These meridians were believed to be interconnected with various organs and bodily functions. By applying pressure to specific points along these meridians, practitioners aimed to restore the flow of qi and promote health.

3. Spreading Across Asia: Acupressure not only thrived in China but also spread to other parts of Asia, including Japan, Korea, and Tibet. Each region developed its own variations and techniques, incorporating acupressure into its traditional healing practices.

4. Integration with Other Healing Systems: Over time, acupressure began to merge with other holistic healing systems, such as Ayurveda in India. This integration enriched the practice and made it even more diverse.

5. Western Recognition: Acupressure gained recognition in the Western world during the 20th century. Books and publications on traditional Chinese medicine, including acupressure, started to circulate, and people in Western countries became more interested in this ancient healing art.

6. Modern Applications: Today, acupressure is widely used as a complementary therapy alongside conventional medical treatments. It is known for its potential benefits in relieving pain, reducing stress, and promoting overall well-being. You can find acupressure practitioners in various parts of the world, offering their services to those seeking natural and holistic healing methods.

The history of acupressure is a testament to the enduring power of ancient healing practices and their ability to adapt and thrive in the modern world. It continues to captivate those seeking a holistic approach to health and wellness, offering a bridge between the past and the present in the realm of complementary and alternative medicine.

2

Chapter 2

Understanding Pressure Points

Locating key pressure points

L ocating key pressure points is a fundamental aspect of acupressure. These points are specific areas on the body where applying pressure can stimulate various physiological and energetic responses. Here are some key pressure points and how to locate them:

1. The Third Eye Point (GV24.5):
   - Location: On the forehead, directly between the eyebrows and slightly above the bridge of the nose.
   - Use: This point is associated with relieving stress, and anxiety, and promoting mental clarity.

2. The Heavenly Pillar (B10):
   - Location: At the base of the skull, on either side of the spine, in the hollows just below the skull's ridge.
   - Use: Massaging these points can help relieve tension in the neck and ease

headaches.

3. The Sea of Tranquility (CV17):
- Location: In the center of the chest, about three finger widths above the base of the breastbone.
- Use: This point is beneficial for calming the mind and reducing anxiety.

4. The Great Rushing (LV3):
- Location: On the top of the foot, between the big and second toes.
- Use: Stimulating this point can help with stress relief and balancing energy flow.

5. The Union Valley (LI4):
- Location: On the back of the hand, in the webbing between the thumb and the index finger.
- Use: This point is famous for relieving pain, especially headaches, and reducing stress.

6. The Pericardium Point (PC6):
- Location: On the inner forearm, about three finger widths up from the wrist crease, between the two tendons.
- Use: It's excellent for reducing anxiety and motion sickness.

7. The Kidney Point (KD27):
- Location: Just below the collarbone, in the hollows on either side of the breastbone.
- Use: This point can help reduce stress and boost energy levels.

8. The Gate of Consciousness (GB20):
- Location: At the base of the skull, in the hollows just behind the ears.
- Use: Massaging these points can alleviate headaches, neck pain, and stress.

To locate these pressure points accurately, use your fingers or thumb, and apply gentle but firm pressure. Start with light pressure and gradually increase it until you feel a mild discomfort or a slight sensation. Remember to take deep breaths and relax when applying pressure. Each of these points serves specific purposes and can be used in acupressure for various conditions, including stress relief, pain management, and overall well-being. Always consult with a trained acupressure practitioner for more specific guidance.

The Meridian System

The meridian system is a fundamental concept in traditional Chinese medicine (TCM) and plays a central role in acupressure and acupuncture. It's an intricate network of energy pathways that run throughout the body, carrying the vital life force known as "qi" (pronounced "chee"). Here's an overview of the meridian system:

1. Channels of Energy: The meridian system consists of a series of channels or pathways through which qi flows. There are 12 primary meridians in the body, each associated with specific organs and functions, such as the liver, heart, lungs, and kidneys.

2. Yin and Yang: Within the meridian system, there is a balance of yin and yang energies. Yin represents the feminine, passive, and receptive energy, while yang is the masculine, active, and dynamic energy. Each meridian is categorized as either yin or yang, and the balance between these energies is crucial for health.

3. Acupressure Points: Along these meridians, there are specific points known as acupressure points or acupuncture points. These points are where acupressure or acupuncture techniques are applied to influence the flow of qi. There are over 300 recognized acupressure points in the body.

4. Balancing Energy: The meridian system is based on the principle that when the flow of qi is balanced and unobstructed, the body is in a state of health and well-being. However, imbalances or blockages in the meridians can lead to various health issues.

5. Diagnosis and Treatment: In traditional Chinese medicine, practitioners diagnose conditions by assessing the flow of qi in the meridians. They use techniques like pulse diagnosis, observation, and patient history to identify imbalances. Treatment methods, including acupressure and acupuncture, aim to restore balance and harmony to the meridian system.

6. Connecting Mind and Body: TCM views the meridian system as a bridge between the physical body and the mind. Emotional and mental well-being is believed to be closely tied to the flow of qi within the meridians. Therefore, acupressure and acupuncture can be used to address not only physical ailments but also emotional and psychological issues.

7. Holistic Approach: The meridian system emphasizes a holistic approach to health, recognizing the interconnectedness of the body's systems and functions. It's not just about treating symptoms but addressing the root causes of health imbalances.

Acupressure, which involves applying pressure to specific acupressure points on the meridians, is designed to influence the flow of qi and promote healing, relaxation, and overall well-being. Understanding the meridian system is crucial for acupressure practitioners as it guides the selection of acupressure points and the development of treatment plans.

3

Chapter 3

Tools and Techniques

Hands and Finger tools

In acupressure, your hands and fingers are your primary tools for applying pressure to specific points on the body. Here's how you can effectively use your hands and fingers as tools for acupressure:

1. Fingers: Your fingers are versatile tools for acupressure. You can use different parts of your fingers to apply pressure to acupressure points, depending on the location and depth required. Here are some finger techniques:

- **Thumb**: The thumb is often used for deep, firm pressure. It's ideal for larger acupressure points or areas that require strong stimulation.

- **Index and Middle Fingers:** These fingers are well-suited for moderate pressure and are often used for points that require precision and accuracy.

- **Tips of Fingers:** The tips of your fingers can be used for very specific and sensitive points that need gentle pressure.

2. Palm: The palm of your hand can be used for broader areas or for gentle, sweeping motions over a series of acupressure points. It's especially useful for promoting relaxation and improving energy flow.

3. Knuckles: The knuckles of your fingers can be used for acupressure points located on the back or areas that require a more extensive surface area for stimulation.

4. Finger Techniques: Various techniques can be applied with your fingers, such as kneading, rotating, and applying steady pressure. You can use the pad of your thumb to press, the sides of your index and middle fingers for sliding or rubbing, and the tips of your fingers for gentle tapping.

5. Using Both Hands: You can use both hands simultaneously to apply pressure to symmetrical points or points on different areas of the body. This can create a balanced and harmonizing effect.

6. Adjusting Pressure: It's essential to communicate with the person receiving acupressure to determine the right level of pressure. You can start with gentle pressure and gradually increase it as needed. The goal is to stimulate the point without causing discomfort or pain.

7. Maintaining Good Posture: When performing acupressure, ensure that you maintain good posture. This helps prevent strain on your hands and fingers and allows you to apply pressure more effectively.

8. Practice and Training: It's beneficial to receive proper training in acupressure techniques to ensure you're applying pressure correctly and targeting the right points. This can help you become more skilled in using your hands and fingers as tools.

Remember that acupressure should be performed with care and precision. Using your hands and fingers as tools allows you to engage with the body's energy meridians and promote well-being by stimulating specific points, relieving tension, and encouraging relaxation.

Other Acupressure tools

In addition to using your hands and fingers, there are various tools and aids that can enhance the practice of acupressure. These tools are designed to provide different sensations and can be especially useful for self-administered acupressure. Here are some common acupressure tools:

1. Acupressure Mats: These mats are covered with numerous small spikes or points that apply pressure to various acupressure points when you lie on them. They are designed to promote relaxation, reduce muscle tension, and alleviate pain.

2. Acupressure Balls and Rollers: These are small, handheld tools with textured surfaces that can be rolled or pressed against acupressure points. They are particularly useful for targeting specific areas, such as the hands, feet, or back.

3. Acupressure Rings: These are metal or plastic rings with small nodules on the inner surface. You can roll them up and down your fingers to stimulate acupressure points on the hands.

4. Acupressure Slippers and Sandals: These footwear items have textured insoles that stimulate acupressure points on the soles of the feet as you walk.

5. Gua Sha Tools: Gua Sha is a traditional Chinese scraping technique used to stimulate blood flow and release tension. Gua Sha tools, often made of jade or other materials, are used to scrape the skin gently along meridian pathways.

6. Electronic Acupressure Devices: These are battery-operated devices that deliver electrical impulses to acupressure points. They are often used for pain relief and muscle relaxation.

7. Acupressure Sticks: These are handheld tools with rounded ends that can be used to apply pressure to specific points, similar to the way your fingers work. They offer a more controlled and consistent pressure.

8. Acupressure Rings for the Ears: These small rings are designed to be worn on the ears and stimulate ear acupressure points. They are used for a wide range of health benefits.

9. Aromatherapy Accessories: Some practitioners combine aromatherapy with acupressure. Essential oils, diffusers, and massage oils can be used to enhance the acupressure experience.

10. Educational Charts and Guides: While not physical tools, charts and guides with detailed acupressure point illustrations and instructions are valuable resources for practitioners and individuals interested in acupressure.

It's important to note that while these tools can complement acupressure practice, they should be used with proper knowledge and guidance. If you are new to acupressure, consider consulting with a trained acupressure practitioner or acupuncturist to learn how to use these tools effectively and safely.

Techniques for effective pressure

Applying the right amount of pressure is crucial for effective acupressure. Here are some techniques for applying pressure effectively when practicing acupressure:

1. Gradual Pressure: Start with light pressure and gradually increase it as needed. This allows the person receiving acupressure to get accustomed to the sensation and helps prevent discomfort.

2. Firm and Steady: Maintain a firm and steady pressure on the acupressure point. Avoid sudden or jerky movements. Steadiness can help the body relax and respond positively to the stimulation.

3. Circular Motion: Use your thumb or fingers to make circular motions on the acupressure point. It is very effective in tension relief. Adjust the size of the circles to match the size of the point.

4. Hold and Release: Apply pressure to the point and hold it for 30 seconds to a minute, or as long as it's comfortable. Then, release the pressure and repeat the process.

5. Rotating Pressure: Apply pressure and gently rotate your thumb or finger in a clockwise or counterclockwise direction. This technique can enhance the stimulation of the point.

6. Pulsing Pressure: Use a pulsing or tapping motion on the acupressure point. This technique is useful for stimulating energy flow and can be less intense than constant pressure.

7. **Breathing in Sync:** Encourage the person receiving acupressure to breathe deeply and in sync with the pressure application. Deep breaths can enhance the relaxation response and help the energy flow.

8. Symmetrical Pressure: If working with paired acupressure points on both sides of the body, apply pressure symmetrically. This helps maintain balance in the body's energy flow.

9. Mindful Focus: Pay attention to the sensation under your fingers and be mindful of any changes in the person's response. This can guide you in adjusting the pressure and technique accordingly.

10. Communication: Continuously communicate with the person receiving acupressure. Ask for feedback on the pressure and whether it feels comfortable or too intense. Everyone's tolerance for pressure varies.

11. Use of Tools: If you're using acupressure tools, follow the instructions provided with the tool and adjust the pressure to the person's comfort.

12. Safety and Caution: Be aware of the contraindications and precautions for specific acupressure points. Some points are not suitable for certain conditions, such as pregnancy, and should be avoided.

Remember that acupressure should be a comfortable and relaxing experience. If there is any pain or discomfort, you should reduce the pressure or discontinue the technique at that particular point. Properly applying these acupressure techniques can help stimulate energy flow, relieve tension, and promote overall well-being.

4

Chapter 4

Ailments and their Acupressure solutions

Headaches: Causes and Acupressure Solutions

Headaches are a common ailment that can range from a mild inconvenience to a debilitating condition. They have various causes, and acupressure can be an effective way to alleviate headache symptoms naturally. Below, we'll explore some common causes of headaches and provide acupressure solutions to help relieve them:

Causes of Headaches:

1. Tension Headaches: These are often caused by muscle tension in the neck and shoulders, stress, and poor posture.

2. Migraines: Migraines are severe headaches often accompanied by symptoms like nausea and sensitivity to light. Their exact cause is not fully understood, but genetics and triggers like certain foods, stress, or hormonal changes can play a role.

3. Sinus Headaches: These occur due to sinus congestion or infections,

leading to pressure and pain in the forehead, cheeks, and eyes.

4. Cluster Headaches: These are intense headaches that occur in clusters or cyclical patterns and are often associated with severe pain around one eye.

5. Dehydration: Lack of proper hydration can lead to headaches.

6. Caffeine Withdrawal: If you're used to regular caffeine intake and suddenly reduce it, withdrawal can result in a headache.

7. Hormonal Changes: Many individuals, especially women, experience headaches related to hormonal fluctuations during menstruation, pregnancy, or menopause.

Acupressure Solutions for Headaches:

1. Third Eye Point:
   - Location: Between the eyebrows, slightly above the bridge of the nose.
   - Acupressure Technique: Gently press this point with your index and middle fingers while taking deep, slow breaths. Hold for 1-2 minutes. This can help alleviate various types of headaches, including tension headaches.

2. Union Valley (LI4):
   - Location: Between the thumb and index finger on the back of the hand.
   - Acupressure Technique: Apply firm pressure and massage this point with your thumb and index finger. Continue for 2-3 minutes. This point is helpful for relieving headache pain, especially migraines.

3. Drilling Bamboo:
   - Location: At the base of the skull, on the back of the head, in line with the top of your ears.
   - Acupressure Technique: Place your thumbs on this point and apply steady, firm pressure. Massage in circular motions for 2-3 minutes. It can help relieve headaches caused by tension and stress.

4. Bright Light:
   - Location: On the forehead, directly above each eyebrow, near the temples.

- Acupressure Technique: Use your index fingers to apply gentle pressure and make small circular movements for 2-3 minutes. This can help with headaches related to sinus congestion.

5. Gates of Consciousness:
   - Location: At the base of the skull, on either side of the spine.
   - Acupressure Technique: Use your thumbs to apply firm pressure to these points. Hold for 2-3 minutes. This can alleviate headaches, including cluster headaches.

6. Lung 2 (LU2):
   - Location: On the upper chest, below the collarbone.
   - Acupressure Technique: Apply gentle pressure to this point with your fingertips. Breathe deeply for 2-3 minutes. It can help with headaches caused by stress and tension.

When using acupressure for headaches, focus on relaxation, deep breathing, and maintaining a comfortable level of pressure. If the headache persists or worsens, it's important to consult a healthcare professional for further evaluation and treatment. Acupressure can be a valuable complementary approach to managing headaches, particularly when used consistently and in conjunction with a healthy lifestyle.

Stress and Anxiety: Causes and Acupressure Solutions

Stress and anxiety are common emotional responses to the demands of daily life, and they can have a significant impact on mental and physical well-being. Acupressure is a natural and effective way to reduce stress and anxiety symptoms. Let's explore some of the causes of stress and anxiety and provide acupressure solutions to help manage these conditions:

Causes of Stress and Anxiety:

1. Work Pressure: High workloads, tight deadlines, and job-related stress can lead to anxiety and tension.

2. Relationship Issues: Conflicts, difficult relationships, or loneliness can contribute to stress and anxiety.

3. Financial Concerns: Worries about money, debts, or financial instability can be a source of chronic stress.

4. Health Concerns: Dealing with illness, chronic pain, or the health of loved ones can trigger anxiety.

5. Trauma: Past traumatic experiences or post-traumatic stress disorder (PTSD) can lead to chronic anxiety.

6. Life Changes: Major life events such as moving, divorce, or the death of a loved one can be stressful and anxiety-inducing.

7. Genetic Predisposition: Some individuals may have a genetic predisposition to anxiety disorders.

Acupressure Solutions for Stress and Anxiety:

1. Sea of Tranquility (CV17):
   - Location: In the center of the chest, about three finger widths above the base of the breastbone.
   - Acupressure Technique: Apply steady pressure to this point with your fingertips. Breathe deeply and hold for 2-3 minutes. It's effective for calming the mind and reducing anxiety.

2. Spirit Gate (HT7):
   - Location: On the wrist, in the depression just below the bone of the pinky

finger.
- Acupressure Technique: Use your thumb to apply gentle pressure to this point for 2-3 minutes. It can help alleviate anxiety and emotional turmoil.

3. Yintang (Extra Point):
- Location: Between the eyebrows, slightly above the bridge of the nose.
- Acupressure Technique: Gently press this point with your index and middle fingers. Hold for 1-2 minutes. It's effective for reducing stress and promoting relaxation.

4. Great Rushing (LV3):
- Location: On the top of the foot, between the big and second toes.
- Acupressure Technique: Apply firm pressure to this point with your thumb for 2-3 minutes. It's beneficial for reducing stress and balancing energy.

5. Inner Gate (PC6):
- Location: On the inner forearm, about three finger widths up from the wrist crease.
- Acupressure Technique: Use your thumb to apply gentle pressure and massage this point for 2-3 minutes. It's helpful for reducing anxiety and calming the heart.

6. Shen Men (HT7):
- Location: On the wrist, in the depression on the pinky side.
- Acupressure Technique: Apply firm pressure with your thumb for 2-3 minutes. It can help relieve anxiety and promote emotional balance.

When using acupressure for stress and anxiety, it's important to focus on deep breathing and relaxation. Maintain a comfortable level of pressure, and you may reduce it if you feel uncomfortable. Acupressure can be a valuable tool for managing stress and anxiety, but it's advisable to consult with a healthcare professional for persistent or severe cases. Combining acupressure with other stress-reduction techniques and a healthy lifestyle can offer comprehensive support for emotional well-being.

Back Pain: Causes and Acupressure Solutions

Back pain is a common condition that can range from mild discomfort to severe debilitation. Acupressure is a natural and effective way to alleviate back pain by targeting specific acupressure points. Let's explore some common causes of back pain and provide acupressure solutions to help manage this condition:

Causes of Back Pain:

1. Muscle Strain: Overexertion, poor posture, or lifting heavy objects can strain the muscles and lead to back pain.

2. Herniated Disc: When the cushioning discs between the vertebrae slip or rupture, it can result in back pain.

3. Spinal Stenosis: A narrowing of the spinal canal can put pressure on the nerves, causing pain.

4. Arthritis: Conditions like osteoarthritis and rheumatoid arthritis can affect the spine and cause pain.

5. Scoliosis: An abnormal curvature of the spine can lead to back discomfort.

6. Sciatica: Pressure on the sciatic nerve can result in radiating pain from the lower back down the leg.

7. Poor Posture: Maintaining an incorrect posture, especially when sitting or standing for extended periods, can contribute to back pain.

Acupressure Solutions for Back Pain:

1. Drilling Bamboo:
   - Location: At the base of the skull, on the back of the head, in line with the top of your ears.

- Acupressure Technique: Place your thumbs on this point and apply steady, firm pressure. Massage in circular motions for 2-3 minutes. It's effective for relieving back pain caused by muscle strain and tension.

2. Gates of Consciousness:
   - Location: At the base of the skull, on either side of the spine.
   - Acupressure Technique: Use your thumbs to apply firm pressure to these points. Hold for 2-3 minutes. It's beneficial for reducing pain in the upper back and neck.

3. Lower Back Points (L1, L2):
   - Location: Find the two points on the lower back, about two inches away from the spine.
   - Acupressure Technique: Apply firm pressure with your thumbs or fingertips to these points for 2-3 minutes. It can help relieve lower back pain.

4. Bladder 23 (BL23):
   - Location: On the lower back, just above the waistline, at the level of the waistband.
   - Acupressure Technique: Use your knuckles to apply firm pressure to this point for 2-3 minutes. It's effective for relieving lower back pain and strengthening the back.

5. Sea of Vitality (B23 and B47):
   - Location: On the back, about two inches away from the spine, at waist level, and just above the waist.
   - Acupressure Technique: Apply firm pressure with your knuckles to these points for 2-3 minutes. It can help alleviate back pain and promote overall vitality.

6. Sacral Points (B48):
   - Location: On the sacrum, in the lower back, just above the buttocks.

- Acupressure Technique: Use your knuckles to apply firm pressure to this point for 2-3 minutes. It's effective for relieving lower back pain and sacral discomfort.

When using acupressure for back pain, maintain a comfortable level of pressure and focus on deep breathing and relaxation. you may reduce it if you feel uncomfortable. Acupressure can be a valuable part of a holistic approach to managing back pain. For chronic or severe cases, it's advisable to consult with a healthcare professional.

Insomnia: Causes and Acupressure Solutions

Insomnia is a frequent sleep condition characterized by difficulties getting asleep, staying asleep, or having poor sleep quality. Acupressure can be a natural and effective way to promote relaxation and improve sleep. Let's explore some common causes of insomnia and provide acupressure solutions to help manage this condition:

Causes of Insomnia:
1. Stress and Anxiety: Persistent worry, stress, and anxiety can make it challenging to relax and fall asleep.
2. Poor Sleep Hygiene: Irregular sleep patterns, excessive screen time before bed, and an uncomfortable sleep environment can contribute to insomnia.
3. Pain or Discomfort: Physical pain, such as back pain or headaches, can disrupt sleep.
4. Medical Conditions: Certain medical conditions, such as sleep apnea or restless leg syndrome, can cause insomnia.
5. Drugs: Certain drugs might disrupt sleep habits.
6. Caffeine and Alcohol: The consumption of caffeine or alcohol close to bedtime can affect sleep.
7. Jet Lag and Shift Work: Rapid time zone changes and irregular work

hours can disrupt the body's internal clock.

Acupressure Solutions for Insomnia:

1. Spirit Gate (HT7):
    - Location: On the wrist, in the depression just below the bone of the pinky finger.
    - Acupressure Technique: Use your thumb to apply gentle pressure to this point for 2-3 minutes. It can help relieve anxiety and promote relaxation for better sleep.

2. YinTang (Extra Point):
    - Location: Between the eyebrows, slightly above the bridge of the nose.
    - Acupressure Technique: Gently press this point with your index and middle fingers. Hold for 1-2 minutes. It's effective for calming the mind and improving sleep quality.

3. Anmian (Extra Point):
    - Location: On the back of the head, about one inch behind the earlobe.
    - Acupressure Technique: Use your fingertips to apply gentle pressure to this point for 2-3 minutes. It can help with insomnia and promote a sense of calm.

4. Shen Men (HT7):
    - Location: On the wrist, in the depression on the pinky side.
    - Acupressure Technique: Apply firm pressure with your thumb for 2-3 minutes. It's beneficial for reducing anxiety and promoting relaxation.

5. Heart 7 (HT7):
    - Location: On the wrist, in line with the little finger and about one inch above the wrist crease.
    - Acupressure Technique: Gently press this point with your thumb for 2-3 minutes to calm the mind and promote sleep.

6. Liver 3 (LR3):
  - Location: On the top of the foot, between the big and second toes.
  - Acupressure Technique: Apply firm pressure with your thumb for 2-3 minutes to reduce stress and promote sleep.

When using acupressure for insomnia, focus on relaxation, deep breathing, and maintaining a comfortable level of pressure. Acupressure can be an effective part of a comprehensive approach to managing insomnia. However, for chronic or severe cases, it's advisable to consult with a healthcare professional for further evaluation and treatment.

Digestive Issues: Causes and Acupressure Solutions

Digestive issues encompass a wide range of problems related to the gastrointestinal system, including indigestion, bloating, constipation, and more. Acupressure can be an effective way to alleviate some of these discomforts. Let's explore common causes of digestive issues and provide acupressure solutions to help manage them:

Causes of Digestive Issues:
  1. Stress and Anxiety: Stress can lead to tension in the gut and disrupt digestion.
  2. Poor Diet: Consuming excessive processed foods, high sugar, and low fiber can result in digestive problems.
  3. Overeating: Large meals or eating too quickly can lead to indigestion.
  4. Food Sensitivities: Some individuals may be sensitive to certain foods, such as dairy or gluten.
  5. Gastroesophageal Reflux Disease (GERD): This condition causes stomach acid to flow back into the esophagus, leading to heartburn and discomfort.
  6. Irritable Bowel Syndrome (IBS): IBS can cause abdominal pain, bloating, and irregular bowel movements.

7. Constipation: Infrequent or difficult bowel movements can lead to discomfort and bloating.

8. Dehydration: Lack of proper hydration can affect digestion and bowel movements.

Acupressure Solutions for Digestive Issues:

1. Pericardium 6 (PC6):
   - Location: On the inner forearm, about three finger widths up from the wrist crease.
   - Acupressure Technique: Use your thumb to apply gentle pressure and massage this point for 2-3 minutes. It can aid with nausea, indigestion, and stomach distress.

2. Stomach 36 (ST36):
   - Location: On the lower leg, about four finger widths below the knee cap and one finger width to the outside of the shin bone.
   - Acupressure Technique: Apply firm pressure to this point with your thumb for 2-3 minutes. It's beneficial for improving overall digestion and reducing bloating.

3. Liver 3 (LR3):
   - Location: On the top of the foot, between the big and second toes.
   - Acupressure Technique: Apply firm pressure with your thumb for 2-3 minutes to relieve abdominal pain and discomfort.

4. Conception Vessel 12 (CV12):
   - Location: In the center of the abdomen, about four finger widths above the navel.
   - Acupressure Technique: Use your fingertips to apply gentle pressure and make small circular movements for 2-3 minutes. This point can alleviate indigestion and bloating.

5. Spleen 6 (SP6):

  - Location: On the inner calf, about four finger widths above the ankle.

  - Acupressure Technique: Apply steady pressure with your thumb for 2-3 minutes. It's effective for promoting healthy digestion and relieving abdominal discomfort.

6. Ren 12 (CV12):

  - Location: In the center of the abdomen, about halfway between the navel and the bottom of the breastbone.

  - Acupressure Technique: Apply gentle pressure with your fingertips and hold for 2-3 minutes to relieve indigestion and discomfort.

When using acupressure for digestive issues, focus on relaxation, deep breathing, and maintaining a comfortable level of pressure. If symptoms persist or worsen, consult with a healthcare professional for further evaluation and treatment. Acupressure can complement other approaches to improving digestive health, such as dietary modifications and lifestyle changes.

Allergies: Causes and Acupressure Solutions

Allergies are the body's immune response to substances that it considers harmful but are generally harmless to others. Common allergy triggers include pollen, dust, pet dander, certain foods, and more. Allergies can cause symptoms like sneezing, runny nose, itching, and congestion. Acupressure can be a natural way to alleviate some of these discomforts. Let's explore common causes of allergies and provide acupressure solutions to help manage them:

Causes of Allergies:

  1. Pollen: Seasonal allergies, also known as hay fever, are often triggered by pollen from trees, grass, and weeds.

2. Dust Mites: These microscopic creatures can be found in dust and are a common indoor allergen.

3. Pet Dander: Allergies to pet dander, which include skin flakes, hair, and saliva, are common among pet owners.

4. Mold Spores: Mold can grow in damp environments and release spores that trigger allergies.

5. Insect Stings: Insect venom from bees, wasps, and other insects can cause allergic reactions.

6. Foods: Allergies to certain foods, such as peanuts, tree nuts, shellfish, and dairy products, can lead to various symptoms.

7. Medications: Allergic reactions can occur as a response to certain medications, like antibiotics or non-steroidal anti-inflammatory drugs.

Acupressure Solutions for Allergies:

1. Welcome Fragrance (LI20):
   - Location: On both sides of the nose, near the nostrils.
   - Acupressure Technique: Use your index fingers to gently press and massage these points for 2-3 minutes. It can help relieve nasal congestion and itching caused by allergies.

2. Heavenly Appearance (LI4):
   - Location: Between the thumb and index finger on the back of the hand.
   - Acupressure Technique: Apply firm pressure and massage this point with your thumb and index finger for 2-3 minutes. It's beneficial for alleviating allergy symptoms, including sneezing.

3. Union Valley (LI4):
   - Location: Between the thumb and index finger on the back of the hand.
   - Acupressure Technique: Apply firm pressure with your thumb for 2-3 minutes. This point can help with allergy symptoms, including itchy eyes and congestion.

4. Drilling Bamboo:
- Location: At the base of the skull, on the back of the head, in line with the top of your ears.
- Acupressure Technique: Place your thumbs on this point and apply steady, firm pressure. Massage in circular motions for 2-3 minutes. It's effective for relieving headaches related to allergies.

5. Welcome Fragrance (Ying Xiang):
- Location: On the sides of the nose, at the level of the nostrils.
- Acupressure Technique: Use your index fingers to apply gentle pressure and massage these points for 2-3 minutes. This can help relieve nasal congestion and sneezing.

6. Wind Screen (GB20):
- Location: At the base of the skull, in the hollows on both sides of the spine.
- Acupressure Technique: Apply gentle pressure with your fingertips for 2-3 minutes. It can help with headaches and eye-related allergy symptoms.

When using acupressure for allergies, focus on relaxation, deep breathing, and maintaining a comfortable level of pressure. Acupressure can be a complementary approach to managing allergy symptoms, but it should be used in conjunction with other allergy management strategies such as avoiding allergens, using medications as prescribed, and consulting with a healthcare professional for severe allergies or anaphylactic reactions.

Nausea: Causes and Acupressure Solutions

Nausea is a common sensation of discomfort in the stomach that often precedes vomiting. It can be caused by various factors, such as motion sickness, morning sickness during pregnancy, gastrointestinal issues, or even stress. Acupressure can be a natural way to relieve nausea and improve overall well-being. Let's explore common causes of nausea and provide acupressure solutions to help manage it:

Causes of Nausea:

1. Motion Sickness: Travel-related motion, such as car, boat, or plane travel, can lead to motion sickness and nausea.

2. Pregnancy: Morning sickness is a common condition during pregnancy, causing nausea.

3. Gastrointestinal Issues: Conditions like indigestion, gastritis, or gastroenteritis can result in nausea.

4. Food Poisoning: Consuming contaminated food or water can lead to nausea and vomiting.

5. Migraines: Some migraines are accompanied by nausea and vomiting.

6. Chemotherapy: Cancer patients undergoing chemotherapy may experience severe nausea.

Acupressure Solutions for Nausea:

1. Pericardium 6 (PC6):
   - Location: On the inner forearm, about three finger widths up from the wrist crease.
   - Acupressure Technique: Use your thumb to apply gentle pressure and massage this point for 2-3 minutes. It's effective for relieving nausea, including motion sickness and morning sickness during pregnancy.

2. Neiguan (PC6):
   - Location: On the inner wrist, about two inches up from the wrist crease, between the tendons.
   - Acupressure Technique: Apply firm pressure with your thumb for 2-3 minutes. It can help with nausea caused by various factors, including motion sickness and gastrointestinal issues.

3. Inner Gate (PC6):

- Location: On the inner forearm, about three finger widths from the wrist crease.
- Acupressure Technique: Use your thumb to apply gentle pressure and massage this point for 2-3 minutes. It can alleviate nausea and improve overall well-being.

4. Stomach 36 (ST36):
   - Location: On the lower leg, about four finger widths below the knee cap and one finger width to the outside of the shin bone.
   - Acupressure Technique: Apply firm pressure with your thumb for 2-3 minutes. This point is effective for relieving nausea and promoting digestion.

5. Ren 12 (CV12):
   - Location: In the center of the abdomen, about four finger widths above the navel.
   - Acupressure Technique: Apply gentle pressure with your fingertips and hold for 2-3 minutes. It can help relieve nausea and discomfort.

6. Sea of Energy (CV6):
   - Location: Two finger widths below the navel, in the center of the abdomen.
   - Acupressure Technique: Use your fingertips to apply gentle pressure and make small circular movements for 2-3 minutes. It's beneficial for relieving nausea and promoting digestion.

When using acupressure for nausea, focus on relaxation, deep breathing, and maintaining a comfortable level of pressure. If nausea persists or worsens, consult with a healthcare professional for further evaluation and treatment. Acupressure can be a valuable complementary approach to managing nausea, particularly when used consistently and in conjunction with other remedies or medications as needed.

Migraines: Causes and Acupressure Solutions

Migraines are severe headaches often accompanied by throbbing pain, sensitivity to light and sound, and nausea. They can significantly impact daily life. Acupressure can be a natural and effective way to alleviate migraine symptoms. Let's explore common causes of migraines and provide acupressure solutions to help manage them:

Causes of Migraines:

1. Genetic Predisposition: Migraines often run in families, suggesting a genetic component.

2. Triggers: Various triggers can lead to migraines, including specific foods, changes in sleep patterns, stress, hormonal fluctuations, and environmental factors.

3. Neurological Changes: Migraines involve changes in brain activity and blood flow, contributing to pain and other symptoms.

4. Hormonal Fluctuations: Some women experience migraines related to hormonal changes during menstruation, pregnancy, or menopause.

5. Sensory Stimuli: Bright lights, loud noises, and strong odors can trigger migraines.

6. Weather Changes: Rapid weather changes or extreme conditions can lead to migraines in some individuals.

Acupressure Solutions for Migraines:

1. Union Valley (LI4):
   - Location: Between the thumb and index finger on the back of the hand.
   - Acupressure Technique: Apply firm pressure with your thumb for 2-3 minutes. This point is effective for relieving migraine pain and promoting relaxation.

2. Third Eye Point (GV24.5):

- Location: In the indentation between the eyebrows, slightly above the bridge of the nose.
- Acupressure Technique: Gently press this point with your index and middle fingers for 1-2 minutes. It can help alleviate migraine pain and reduce sensitivity to light.

3. Drilling Bamboo (B2):
- Location: At the base of the skull, on the back of the head, in line with the top of your ears.
- Acupressure Technique: Place your thumbs on this point and apply steady, firm pressure. Massage in circular motions for 2-3 minutes. It can help relieve migraine pain and tension.

4. Gates of Consciousness (GV20):
- Location: At the top of the head, along the midline.
- Acupressure Technique: Use your fingertips to apply gentle pressure for 2-3 minutes. It can alleviate migraine pain and promote relaxation.

5. Great Eliminator (LV3):
- Location: On the top of the foot, between the big and second toes.
- Acupressure Technique: Apply firm pressure with your thumb for 2-3 minutes. It's beneficial for relieving migraine pain and promoting overall well-being.

6. Large Intestine 10 (LI10):
- Location: On the forearm, about two thumb widths below the elbow crease.
- Acupressure Technique: Use your thumb to apply firm pressure and massage this point for 2-3 minutes. It can help reduce migraine pain and tension.

When using acupressure for migraines, focus on relaxation, deep breathing, and maintaining a comfortable level of pressure. If migraines persist or worsen, consult with a healthcare professional for further evaluation and treatment. Acupressure can be a valuable complementary approach to managing migraines, especially when used consistently and in conjunction with other migraine management strategies.

Sinus Congestion: Causes and Acupressure Solutions

Sinus congestion, often accompanied by symptoms like a stuffy or runny nose, facial pain, and pressure, can be caused by various factors, including allergies, infections, and environmental irritants. Acupressure can be a natural and effective way to relieve sinus congestion and improve breathing. Let's explore common causes of sinus congestion and provide acupressure solutions to help manage it:

Causes of Sinus Congestion:

1. Allergies: Allergic reactions to pollen, dust, pet dander, and other allergens can lead to sinus congestion.

2. Infections: Viral or bacterial infections, such as the common cold or sinusitis, can cause sinus congestion.

3. Environmental Irritants: Exposure to smoke, pollution, or other irritants can irritate the sinuses and lead to congestion.

4. Structural Issues: Deviated septum, nasal polyps, or other structural problems in the nasal passages can contribute to sinus congestion.

5. Dry Air: Low humidity levels can dry out the nasal passages, making them more prone to congestion.

6. Changes in Weather: Sudden temperature or pressure changes can trigger sinus congestion in some individuals.

Acupressure Solutions for Sinus Congestion:

1. Welcome Fragrance (LI20):

- Location: On both sides of the nose, near the nostrils.
- Acupressure Technique: Use your index fingers to gently press and massage these points for 2-3 minutes. It can help relieve nasal congestion and sinus pressure.

2. Bright Light (ST1):
   - Location: On the lower edge of the eye socket, just below the pupil.
   - Acupressure Technique: Apply gentle pressure to this point with your index fingers for 2-3 minutes. It's beneficial for relieving sinus congestion and eye-related symptoms.

3. Drilling Bamboo (B2):
   - Location: At the base of the skull, on the back of the head, in line with the top of your ears.
   - Acupressure Technique: Place your thumbs on this point and apply steady, firm pressure. Massage in circular motions for 2-3 minutes. It can help reduce nasal congestion and encourage relaxation.

4. Welcome Fragrance (Ying Xiang):
   - Location: On the sides of the nose, at the level of the nostrils.
   - Acupressure Technique: Use your index fingers to apply gentle pressure and make small circular movements for 2-3 minutes. This can help relieve nasal congestion and sinus pressure.

5. Bitong (GV20):
   - Location: At the top of the head, along the midline.
   - Acupressure Technique: Use your fingertips to apply gentle pressure for 2-3 minutes. It can alleviate sinus congestion and promote overall well-being.

6. Yangbai (GB14):
   - Location: On the forehead, about one inch above the center of each eyebrow.
   - Acupressure Technique: Apply gentle pressure to this point with your

fingertips for 2-3 minutes. It can help with sinus congestion and promote relaxation.

When using acupressure for sinus congestion, focus on relaxation, deep breathing, and maintaining a comfortable level of pressure. If congestion persists or worsens, consult with a healthcare professional for further evaluation and treatment. Acupressure can be a valuable complementary approach to managing sinus congestion, particularly when used consistently and in conjunction with other remedies or medications as needed.

Neck Pain: Causes and Acupressure Solutions

Neck pain is a common discomfort that can range from mild to severe and often results from issues like muscle strain, poor posture, or underlying medical conditions. Acupressure can be a natural and effective way to alleviate neck pain by targeting specific acupressure points. Let's explore common causes of neck pain and provide acupressure solutions to help manage it:

Causes of Neck Pain:
1. Muscle Strain: Overuse, poor posture, or sudden movements can strain the neck muscles, leading to pain.
2. Poor Posture: Maintaining an incorrect posture, especially when sitting or standing for extended periods, can contribute to neck pain.
3. Cervical Spondylosis: Age-related wear and tear can lead to neck pain and stiffness.
4. Injury: Accidents or trauma can result in neck pain, including whiplash.
5. Herniated Disc: A herniated cervical disc can press on nerves, causing neck pain.
6. Arthritis: Conditions like osteoarthritis and rheumatoid arthritis can affect the neck and cause pain.
7. Stress and Tension: Emotional stress can lead to tension in the neck and

shoulder muscles.

Acupressure Solutions for Neck Pain:

1. Gates of Consciousness (GB20):
   - Location: At the base of the skull, in the hollows on both sides of the spine.
   - Acupressure Technique: Use your fingertips to apply gentle pressure for 2-3 minutes. This point is effective for relieving neck pain and tension.

2. Heavenly Pillar (B10):
   - Location: On either side of the spine, in the hollows below the base of the skull.
   - Acupressure Technique: Apply gentle pressure with your fingertips for 2-3 minutes. It can help alleviate neck pain and promote relaxation.

3. Wind Pool (GB20):
   - Location: On the back of the neck, about two finger widths below the base of the skull.
   - Acupressure Technique: Use your fingertips to apply firm pressure for 2-3 minutes. It's beneficial for relieving neck pain and tension.

4. Large Intestine 4 (LI4):
   - Location: Between the thumb and index finger on the back of the hand.
   - Acupressure Technique: Apply firm pressure and massage this point with your thumb and index finger for 2-3 minutes. It can help alleviate neck pain and tension.

5. Three Mile Point (ST36):
   - Location: On the lower leg, about four finger widths below the knee cap and one finger width to the outside of the shin bone.
   - Acupressure Technique: Apply firm pressure with your thumb for 2-3 minutes. This point is effective for reducing neck pain and promoting overall

relaxation.

6. Drilling Bamboo (B2):
   - Location: At the base of the skull, on the back of the head, in line with the top of your ears.
   - Acupressure Technique: Place your thumbs on this point and apply steady, firm pressure. Massage in circular motions for 2-3 minutes. Effective in tension and pain relief.

When using acupressure for neck pain, focus on relaxation, deep breathing, and maintaining a comfortable level of pressure. If neck pain persists or worsens, consult with a healthcare professional for further evaluation and treatment. Acupressure can be a valuable part of a holistic approach to managing neck pain, particularly when used consistently and in conjunction with other remedies or therapies as needed.

Shoulder Tension: Causes and Acupressure Solutions

Shoulder tension is a common issue that can result from stress, poor posture, overuse, or underlying muscular problems. Acupressure can be a natural and effective way to alleviate shoulder tension by targeting specific acupressure points. Let's explore common causes of shoulder tension and provide acupressure solutions to help manage it:

Causes of Shoulder Tension:
   1. Stress and Anxiety: Emotional stress can lead to muscle tension in the shoulders.
   2. Poor Posture: Maintaining an incorrect posture, especially when sitting at a desk or using electronic devices, can contribute to shoulder tension.
   3. Overuse: Repetitive movements or overusing the shoulder muscles can result in tension.
   4. Muscle Imbalance: Imbalances in the shoulder muscles can lead to

tension and discomfort.

5. Injury: Trauma or injuries to the shoulder area can cause ongoing tension.

6. Sleep Position: Sleeping in an uncomfortable position can lead to morning shoulder tension.

Acupressure Solutions for Shoulder Tension:

1. Gallbladder 21 (GB21):
   - Location: On the top of the shoulder, halfway between the base of the neck and the tip of the shoulder.
   - Acupressure Technique: Use your fingertips to apply firm pressure for 2-3 minutes. This point is effective for relieving shoulder tension.

2. Shoulder Well (LI15):
   - Location: On the outer shoulder, in a small depression between the end of the collarbone and the shoulder joint.
   - Acupressure Technique: Apply firm pressure with your fingertips for 2-3 minutes. It can help alleviate shoulder tension and discomfort.

3. Heavenly Pillar (B10):
   - Location: On the back of the neck, on either side of the spine, in the hollows below the base of the skull.
   - Acupressure Technique: Apply gentle pressure with your fingertips for 2-3 minutes. It's beneficial for relieving shoulder tension and promoting relaxation.

4. Gates of Consciousness (GB20):
   - Location: At the base of the skull, in the hollows on both sides of the spine.
   - Acupressure Technique: Use your fingertips to apply gentle pressure for 2-3 minutes. This point is effective for relieving shoulder tension and promoting relaxation.

5. Large Intestine 4 (LI4):

   - Location: Between the thumb and index finger on the back of the hand.

   - Acupressure Technique: Apply firm pressure and massage this point with your thumb and index finger for 2-3 minutes. It can help alleviate shoulder tension and promote relaxation.

6. Triple Burner 5 (TB5):

   - Location: On the outer side of the forearm, about two inches above the wrist crease.

   - Acupressure Technique: Apply firm pressure with your fingertips for 2-3 minutes. It's beneficial for reducing shoulder tension and promoting overall relaxation.

When using acupressure for shoulder tension, focus on relaxation, deep breathing, and maintaining a comfortable level of pressure. If shoulder tension persists or worsens, consult with a healthcare professional for further evaluation and treatment. Acupressure can be a valuable part of a holistic approach to managing shoulder tension, particularly when used consistently and in conjunction with other remedies or therapies as needed.

High Blood Pressure: Causes and Acupressure Solutions

High blood pressure, commonly known as hypertension, is a medical condition in which the force of blood against the artery walls is constantly too great. If not addressed, it can lead to major health problems. Acupressure can complement other approaches to managing blood pressure, such as medication and lifestyle changes. Let's explore common causes of high blood pressure and provide acupressure solutions to help manage it:

Causes of High Blood Pressure:

   1. Lifestyle Factors: Unhealthy eating habits, lack of physical activity,

smoking, and excessive alcohol consumption can contribute to high blood pressure.

2. Genetics: Family history can play a role in hypertension.

3. Stress: Chronic stress can lead to elevated blood pressure levels.

4. Obesity: Excess body weight can strain the cardiovascular system and increase blood pressure.

5. Chronic Kidney Disease: Kidney problems can impact blood pressure regulation.

6. Hormonal Conditions: Conditions like hyperthyroidism or adrenal gland disorders can lead to high blood pressure.

Acupressure Solutions for High Blood Pressure:

1. Union Valley (LI4):
   - Location: Between the thumb and index finger on the back of the hand.
   - Acupressure Technique: Apply firm pressure and massage this point with your thumb and index finger for 2-3 minutes. It can help promote relaxation and reduce blood pressure.

2. Pericardium 6 (PC6):
   - Location: On the inner forearm, about three finger widths up from the wrist crease.
   - Acupressure Technique: Use your thumb to apply gentle pressure and massage this point for 2-3 minutes. It has the potential to lower blood pressure and induce relaxation.

3. Kidney 1 (KD1):
   - Location: On the sole of the foot, in the depression at the center of the sole.
   - Acupressure Technique: Apply gentle pressure with your thumb for 2-3 minutes. This point can help balance kidney function, which plays a role in blood pressure regulation.

4. Yintang (Extra Point):
  - Location: Between the eyebrows, slightly above the bridge of the nose.
  - Acupressure Technique: Gently press this point with your index and middle fingers. Hold for 1-2 minutes. It can help with blood pressure regulation and relaxation.

5. Heart 7 (HT7):
  - Location: On the wrist, in line with the little finger and about one inch above the wrist crease.
  - Acupressure Technique: Gently press this point with your thumb for 2-3 minutes to promote relaxation and reduce blood pressure.

6. Spleen 6 (SP6):
  - Location: On the inner calf, about four finger widths above the ankle.
  - Acupressure Technique: Apply steady pressure with your thumb for 2-3 minutes. It can help with blood pressure regulation and overall well-being.

When using acupressure for high blood pressure, focus on relaxation, deep breathing, and maintaining a comfortable level of pressure. Acupressure can be a complementary approach to managing high blood pressure, but it should not replace medical treatment or lifestyle changes when necessary. If you have high blood pressure, consult with a healthcare professional for a comprehensive evaluation and management plan.

Low Energy: Causes and Acupressure Solutions

Low energy, often accompanied by feelings of fatigue and sluggishness, can result from various factors, including lifestyle, sleep patterns, and stress. Acupressure can be a natural and effective way to boost energy levels and improve overall vitality. Let's explore common causes of low energy and provide acupressure solutions to help manage it:

Causes of Low Energy:

1. Poor Sleep: Inadequate or disrupted sleep can lead to low energy levels.

2. Stress and Anxiety: Chronic stress and anxiety can drain your energy.

3. Diet and Nutrition: An unhealthy diet or skipping meals can result in low energy.

4. Dehydration: Inadequate hydration can cause feelings of fatigue.

5. Lack of Physical Activity: A sedentary lifestyle can lead to low energy levels.

6. Medical Conditions: Conditions like anemia, thyroid disorders, and chronic fatigue syndrome can cause persistent low energy.

Acupressure Solutions for Low Energy:

1. Sea of Energy (CV6):
   - Location: Two finger widths below the navel, in the center of the abdomen.
   - Acupressure Technique: Use your fingertips to apply gentle pressure and make small circular movements for 2-3 minutes. It can help boost energy and vitality.

2. Gates of Consciousness (GB20):
   - Location: At the base of the skull, in the hollows on both sides of the spine.
   - Acupressure Technique: Use your fingertips to apply gentle pressure for 2-3 minutes. This point can alleviate feelings of fatigue and promote relaxation.

3. Yongquan (KI1):
   - Location: On the sole of the foot, in the depression at the center of the heel.
   - Acupressure Technique: Apply gentle pressure with your thumb for 2-3 minutes. This point can help revitalize your energy and improve your overall well-being.

4. Three Mile Point (ST36):
   - Location: On the lower leg, about four finger widths below the knee cap and one finger width to the outside of the shin bone.
   - Acupressure Technique: Apply firm pressure with your thumb for 2-3 minutes. This point is effective for boosting energy and promoting vitality.

5. Spleen 6 (SP6):
   - Location: On the inner calf, about four finger widths above the ankle.
   - Acupressure Technique: Apply steady pressure with your thumb for 2-3 minutes. It can help improve energy levels and overall well-being.

6. Conception Vessel 6 (CV6):
   -Location: Close to two fingers wide below the navel region.
   - Acupressure Technique: Use your fingertips to apply gentle pressure and make small circular movements for 2-3 minutes. This point can help boost energy and vitality.

When using acupressure for low energy, focus on relaxation, deep breathing, and maintaining a comfortable level of pressure. If low energy persists or worsens, consult with a healthcare professional to rule out underlying medical conditions. Acupressure can be a valuable part of a holistic approach to boosting energy levels, particularly when used consistently and in conjunction with other lifestyle adjustments.

Menstrual Cramps: Causes and Acupressure Solutions

Dysmenorrhea, also known as menstrual cramps is a frequent discomfort that many women feel during their menstrual cycle.. These cramps can range from mild to severe and are typically caused by uterine contractions. Acupressure can provide natural relief from menstrual cramps by targeting specific acupressure points. Let's explore common causes of menstrual cramps and provide acupressure solutions to help manage them:

Causes of Menstrual Cramps:

1. Uterine Contractions: The uterus contracts to shed its lining, leading to cramps.

2. Prostaglandins: The release of prostaglandins, hormone-like substances, can cause more intense contractions and pain.

3. Fibroids and Endometriosis: Conditions like fibroids or endometriosis can lead to more severe menstrual cramps.

4. Heavy Menstrual Flow: Excessive bleeding during the menstrual period can result in stronger cramps.

5. Emotional Factors: Stress and anxiety can worsen menstrual cramps.

Acupressure Solutions for Menstrual Cramps:

1. Spleen 6 (SP6):
  - Location: On the inner calf, about four finger widths above the ankle.
  - Acupressure Technique: Apply steady pressure with your thumb for 2-3 minutes. This point can help relieve menstrual cramps and improve overall well-being.

2. Lower Abdomen (CV4):
  -Location: Close to two fingers wide below the navel region.
  - Acupressure Technique: Use your fingertips to apply gentle pressure and make small circular movements for 2-3 minutes. It can help alleviate menstrual cramps and discomfort.

3. San Yin Jiao (SP6):
  - Location: On the inner calf, about four finger widths above the ankle.
  - Acupressure Technique: Apply steady pressure with your thumb for 2-3 minutes. This point is effective for relieving menstrual cramps and promoting relaxation.

4. Conception Vessel 4 (CV4):
  -Location: Close to two fingers wide below the navel region.
  - Acupressure Technique: Use your fingertips to apply gentle pressure and make small circular movements for 2-3 minutes. It can aid in the relief of menstrual cramps and pain.

5. Sacral Points (Sacrum):
  - Location: In the lower back, along the sacrum, about two inches above the tailbone.
  - Acupressure Technique: Apply gentle pressure with your fingertips for 2-3 minutes. It can help alleviate lower back pain often associated with menstrual cramps.

6. Liver 3 (LR3):
  - Location: On the top of the foot, between the big and second toes.
  - Acupressure Technique: Apply firm pressure with your thumb for 2-3 minutes. This point can help reduce pain and discomfort associated with menstrual cramps.

When using acupressure for menstrual cramps, focus on relaxation, deep breathing, and maintaining a comfortable level of pressure. If menstrual cramps are severe or persistent, consult with a healthcare professional for further evaluation and treatment. Acupressure can be a valuable complementary approach to managing menstrual cramps, particularly when used consistently and in conjunction with other remedies or therapies as needed.

Lower Back Pain: Causes and Acupressure Solutions

Lower back pain is a common issue that can result from various factors, including muscle strain, poor posture, or underlying medical conditions.

Acupressure can be a natural and effective way to alleviate lower back pain by targeting specific acupressure points. Let's explore common causes of lower back pain and provide acupressure solutions to help manage it:

Causes of Lower Back Pain:

1. Muscle Strain: Overuse, lifting heavy objects, or sudden movements can strain the lower back muscles, leading to pain.

2. Poor Posture: Maintaining an incorrect posture, especially when sitting for extended periods, can contribute to lower back pain.

3. Herniated Disc: A herniated disc can press on nerves in the lower back, causing pain.

4. Arthritis: Conditions like osteoarthritis and ankylosing spondylitis can affect the lower back and cause pain.

5. Injury: Trauma or accidents can result in lower back pain, including whiplash injuries.

6. Spinal Stenosis: Narrowing of the spinal canal can lead to lower back pain.

Acupressure Solutions for Lower Back Pain:

1. Governing Vessel 20 (GV20):
   - Location: At the top of the head, along the midline.
   - Acupressure Technique: Use your fingertips to apply gentle pressure for 2-3 minutes. This point can help alleviate lower back pain and promote relaxation.

2. Bladder 23 (BL23):
   - Location: On the lower back, about one-and-a-half inches on each side of the spine, at waist level.
   - Acupressure Technique: Apply firm pressure with your fingertips for 2-3 minutes. This point is effective for relieving lower back pain and discomfort.

3. Bladder 40 (BL40):

- Location: On the back of the leg, about two finger widths above the back of the knee crease.
- Acupressure Technique: Apply firm pressure with your thumb for 2-3 minutes. This point can help alleviate lower back pain and promote relaxation.

4. Sacrum Points (Sacrum):
   - Location: In the lower back, along the sacrum, about two inches above the tailbone.
   - Acupressure Technique: Apply gentle pressure with your fingertips for 2-3 minutes. These points can help relieve lower back pain and discomfort.

5. Bladder 62 (BL62):
   - Location: On the top of the foot, at the depression between the fourth and fifth metatarsal bones.
   - Acupressure Technique: Apply firm pressure with your thumb for 2-3 minutes. This point can help reduce lower back pain and promote overall well-being.

6. Triple Burner 3 (TB3):
   - Location: On the back of the hand, between the fourth and fifth metacarpal bones, at the level of the knuckles.
   - Acupressure Technique: Apply firm pressure with your thumb for 2-3 minutes. This point is effective for relieving lower back pain and promoting relaxation.

When using acupressure for lower back pain, focus on relaxation, deep breathing, and maintaining a

comfortable level of pressure. If lower back pain persists or worsens, consult with a healthcare professional for further evaluation and treatment. Acupressure can be a valuable part of a holistic approach to managing lower back pain, particularly when used consistently and in conjunction with other remedies or therapies as needed.

Respiratory Issues: Causes and Acupressure Solutions

Respiratory issues can encompass a range of conditions affecting the lungs and airways, including conditions like asthma, bronchitis, and allergies. Acupressure can provide relief for some respiratory symptoms and help improve lung function. Let's explore common causes of respiratory issues and provide acupressure solutions to help manage them:

Causes of Respiratory Issues:

1. Asthma: An inflammatory condition that narrows the airways, making breathing difficult.

2. Bronchitis: Inflammation of the bronchial tubes, often due to viral or bacterial infections.

3. Allergies: Allergic reactions to pollen, dust, pet dander, or other allergens can trigger respiratory symptoms.

4. Chronic Obstructive Pulmonary Disease (COPD): A progressive lung disease that includes chronic bronchitis and emphysema.

5. Respiratory Infections: Infections like the common cold or flu can lead to respiratory symptoms.

6. Environmental Irritants: Exposure to smoke, pollution, or other irritants can aggravate respiratory conditions.

Acupressure Solutions for Respiratory Issues:

1. Lung 9 (LU9):
   - Location: On the wrist, in line with the thumb, at the crease of the wrist.
   - Acupressure Technique: Use your thumb to apply gentle pressure for 2-3 minutes. This point can help with respiratory issues and promote lung health.

2. Lung 7 (LU7):
  - Location: On the arm, about two finger widths above the wrist crease.
  - Acupressure Technique: Apply gentle pressure with your thumb for 2-3 minutes. It can help with respiratory symptoms and improve lung function.

3. Large Intestine 4 (LI4):
  - Location: Between the thumb and index finger on the back of the hand.
  - Acupressure Technique: Apply firm pressure and massage this point with your thumb and index finger for 2-3 minutes. It can help with respiratory issues and promote relaxation.

4. Conception Vessel 17 (CV17):
  - Location: In the center of the chest, at the level of the fourth intercostal space (between the ribs).
  - Acupressure Technique: Use your fingertips to apply gentle pressure for 2-3 minutes. This point can help with respiratory symptoms and promote lung health.

5. Acupressure for Acupuncture Point Lung 1 (LU1):
  - Location: On the upper chest, about one inch below the collarbone.
  - Acupressure Technique: Apply gentle pressure with your fingertips for 2-3 minutes. It can help with respiratory issues and promote relaxation.

6. Conception Vessel 22 (CV22):
  - Location: At the base of the throat, in the notch at the top of the sternum.
  - Acupressure Technique: Use your fingertips to apply gentle pressure for 2-3 minutes. It can help relieve respiratory symptoms and promote lung health.

When using acupressure for respiratory issues, focus on relaxation, deep breathing, and maintaining a comfortable level of pressure. It's important to consult with a healthcare professional for proper diagnosis and treatment of respiratory conditions. Acupressure can be a valuable complementary approach to managing respiratory symptoms, particularly when used consistently and in conjunction with other remedies or therapies as recommended by a healthcare provider.

Jaw Pain: Causes and Acupressure Solutions

Jaw pain, often associated with conditions like temporomandibular joint (TMJ) disorder, can be a source of discomfort and may result from various factors, including muscle tension, dental issues, or stress. Acupressure can provide relief for jaw pain by targeting specific acupressure points. Let's explore common causes of jaw pain and provide acupressure solutions to help manage it:

Causes of Jaw Pain:

1. Temporomandibular Joint (TMJ) Disorder: Dysfunction of the TMJ can lead to jaw pain, clicking, and difficulty opening or closing the mouth.

2. Bruxism (Teeth Grinding): Clenching or grinding the teeth, often during sleep, can result in jaw pain.

3. Dental Issues: Problems with the teeth, such as misalignment or dental work, can contribute to jaw pain.

4. Stress and Tension: Emotional stress can cause jaw muscle tension and pain.

5. Arthritis: Conditions like osteoarthritis can affect the jaw joint and lead to pain.

6. Injury: Trauma to the jaw, such as a blow or impact, can result in jaw pain.

Acupressure Solutions for Jaw Pain:

1. Jaw Acupressure Point (Stomach 7 - ST7):
   - Location: On the jawline, directly in front of the earlobe.

- Acupressure Technique: Use your fingertips to apply gentle pressure for 2-3 minutes. This point can help alleviate jaw pain and promote relaxation.

2. Large Intestine 4 (LI4):
   - Location: Between the thumb and index finger on the back of the hand.
   - Acupressure Technique: Apply firm pressure and massage this point with your thumb and index finger for 2-3 minutes. It can help with jaw pain and reduce muscle tension.

3. Stomach 6 (ST6):
   - Location: In the hollow below the cheekbone, in line with the edge of the nostril.
   - Acupressure Technique: Apply gentle pressure with your fingertips for 2-3 minutes. This point can help relieve jaw pain and discomfort.

4. Gallbladder 20 (GB20):
   - Location: At the base of the skull, in the hollows on both sides of the spine.
   - Acupressure Technique: Use your fingertips to apply gentle pressure for 2-3 minutes. This point can help alleviate jaw pain and promote relaxation.

5. Triple Burner 23 (TB23):
   - Location: At the outer end of the eyebrow, directly above the outer corner of the eye.
   - Acupressure Technique: Apply gentle pressure with your fingertips for 2-3 minutes. It can help with jaw pain and promote relaxation.

6. Large Intestine 18 (LI18):
   - Location: Just below the cheekbone, in line with the outside corner of the eye.
   - Acupressure Technique: Apply gentle pressure with your fingertips for 2-3 minutes. Very effective in the reduction of jaw discomfort or pain.

When using acupressure for jaw pain, focus on relaxation, deep breathing, and maintaining a comfortable level of pressure. If jaw pain persists or worsens, consult with a healthcare professional or a dentist for proper evaluation and treatment. Acupressure can be a valuable complementary approach to managing jaw pain, particularly when used consistently and in conjunction with other remedies or therapies as recommended by a healthcare provider.

Chest Congestion: Causes and Acupressure Solutions

Chest congestion is a common issue that can result from various factors, including respiratory infections, allergies, or environmental irritants. It often leads to discomfort, difficulty breathing, and a feeling of heaviness in the chest. Acupressure can provide relief for chest congestion by targeting specific acupressure points. Let's explore common causes of chest congestion and provide acupressure solutions to help manage it:

Causes of Chest Congestion:
1. Respiratory Infections: Viral or bacterial infections, such as the common cold or bronchitis, can lead to chest congestion.
2. Allergies: Allergic reactions to pollen, dust, pet dander, or other allergens can trigger chest congestion.
3. Environmental Irritants: Exposure to smoke, pollution, or other irritants can aggravate chest congestion.
4. Asthma: Asthma can cause inflammation and mucus production, leading to chest congestion.
5. Chronic Obstructive Pulmonary Disease (COPD): A progressive lung disease that includes chronic bronchitis and emphysema can result in chest congestion.

Acupressure Solutions for Chest Congestion:

1. Lung 1 (LU1):
   - Location: On the upper chest, about one inch below the collarbone.
   - Acupressure Technique: Use your fingertips to apply gentle pressure for 2-3 minutes. This point can help relieve chest congestion and promote easier breathing.

2. Lung 9 (LU9):
   - Location: On the wrist, in line with the thumb, at the crease of the wrist.
   - Acupressure Technique: Use your thumb to apply gentle pressure for 2-3 minutes. This point can help with chest congestion and promote lung health.

3. Ren 17 (CV17):
   - Location: In the center of the chest, at the level of the fourth intercostal space (between the ribs).
   - Acupressure Technique: Use your fingertips to apply gentle pressure for 2-3 minutes. This point can help relieve chest congestion and promote easier breathing.

4. Conception Vessel 22 (CV22):
   - Location: At the base of the throat, in the notch at the top of the sternum.
   - Acupressure Technique: Use your fingertips to apply gentle pressure for 2-3 minutes. This point can help relieve chest congestion and promote easier breathing.

5. Gallbladder 21 (GB21):
   - Location: At the top of the shoulder, along the edge of the shoulder muscle.
   - Acupressure Technique: Use your fingertips to apply gentle pressure for 2-3 minutes. This point can help relieve chest congestion and promote relaxation.

6. Stomach 40 (ST40):
   - Location: On the front of the leg, about three finger widths below the knee cap.

- Acupressure Technique: Apply gentle pressure with your fingertips for 2-3 minutes. This point can help reduce chest congestion and improve overall well-being.

When using acupressure for chest congestion, focus on relaxation, deep breathing, and maintaining a comfortable level of pressure. It's important to consult with a healthcare professional for proper diagnosis and treatment of chest congestion, especially if it's due to an underlying condition. Acupressure can be a valuable complementary approach to managing chest congestion, particularly when used consistently and in conjunction with other remedies or therapies as recommended by a healthcare provider.

Motion Sickness: Causes and Acupressure Solutions

Motion sickness is a common condition that occurs when your brain receives mixed signals from your inner ears, eyes, and sensory receptors, usually due to motion, such as in a car, boat, or airplane. This mismatch of sensory information can lead to symptoms like nausea, dizziness, and vomiting. Acupressure can provide relief from motion sickness by targeting specific acupressure points. Let's explore common causes of motion sickness and provide acupressure solutions to help manage it:

Causes of Motion Sickness:
1. Sensory Mismatch: When the signals from your inner ears, eyes, and other sensory receptors don't match, it can lead to motion sickness.
2. Travel and Motion: Traveling in cars, boats, planes, or other modes of transportation can trigger motion sickness.
3. Reading in Motion: Reading or looking at screens while in motion can exacerbate symptoms.
4. Stress and Anxiety: Emotional factors can contribute to motion sickness.
5. Individual Sensitivity: Some people are more prone to motion sickness

than others.

Acupressure Solutions for Motion Sickness:

1. Pericardium 6 (PC6):
   - Location: On the inner forearm, about three finger widths up from the wrist crease.
   - Acupressure Technique: Use your thumb to apply gentle pressure and massage this point for 2-3 minutes. This point is well-known for relieving nausea and motion sickness.

2. Stomach 36 (ST36):
   - Location: On the lower leg, about four finger widths below the knee cap and one finger width to the outside of the shin bone.
   - Acupressure Technique: Apply gentle pressure with your thumb for 2-3 minutes. This point can help reduce nausea and dizziness associated with motion sickness.

3. Gallbladder 20 (GB20):
   - Location: At the base of the skull, in the hollows on both sides of the spine.
   - Acupressure Technique: Use your fingertips to apply gentle pressure for 2-3 minutes. This point is effective for relieving motion sickness and dizziness.

4. Conception Vessel 6 (CV6):
   - Location: Close to two fingers wide below the navel region.
   - Acupressure Technique: Use your fingertips to apply gentle pressure and make small circular movements for 2-3 minutes. This point can help reduce nausea and discomfort associated with motion sickness.

5. Liver 3 (LR3):
   - Location: On the top of the foot, between the big and second toes.

- Acupressure Technique: Apply gentle pressure for 2-3 minutes. This point can help with motion sickness and promote relaxation.

6. Large Intestine 4 (LI4):
   - Location: Between the thumb and index finger on the back of the hand.
   - Acupressure Technique: Apply firm pressure and massage this point with your thumb and index finger for 2-3 minutes. It can help relieve motion sickness symptoms.

When using acupressure for motion sickness, focus on relaxation, deep breathing, and maintaining a comfortable level of pressure. It's also helpful to look out at the horizon or a fixed point to help align sensory information. If motion sickness is a recurrent issue, consider other remedies, such as medication or avoiding triggers, and consult with a healthcare professional for guidance. Acupressure can be a valuable complementary approach to managing motion sickness, particularly when used consistently and in conjunction with other strategies.

Depression: Causes and Acupressure Solutions

Depression is a complicated mental health illness characterized by persistent feelings of sorrow, despair, and a loss of interest in activities. While acupressure can provide some relief from symptoms and stress associated with depression, it should not replace professional treatment for clinical depression. Always consult with a mental health professional for a comprehensive evaluation and appropriate treatment. Acupressure can be a complementary approach to help manage stress and promote relaxation. Let's explore common causes of depression and provide acupressure solutions for stress relief:

Causes of Depression:

1. Biological Factors: Imbalances in brain chemicals, genetics, and hormonal changes can contribute to depression.

2. Psychological Factors: Past trauma, negative thought patterns, and self-esteem issues can play a role in depression.

3. Environmental Factors: Chronic stress, isolation, and major life events can trigger or worsen depressive symptoms.

4. Medical Conditions: Certain medical conditions and medications can be associated with depression.

Acupressure Solutions for Stress Relief:

1. Pericardium 6 (PC6):
   - Location: On the inner forearm, about three finger widths up from the wrist crease.
   - Acupressure Technique: Use your thumb to apply gentle pressure and massage this point for 2-3 minutes. This spot is well-known for relieving tension and anxiety.

2. Conception Vessel 17 (CV17):
   - Location: In the center of the chest, at the level of the fourth intercostal space (between the ribs).
   - Acupressure Technique: Use your fingertips to apply gentle pressure for 2-3 minutes. This point can help alleviate stress and promote relaxation.

3. Governing Vessel 24.5 (GV24.5):
   - Location: At the point between the eyebrows, slightly above the bridge of the nose.
   - Acupressure Technique: Gently press this point with your index and middle fingers. Hold for 1-2 minutes. It can assist to alleviate tension and soothe the mind.

4. Liver 3 (LR3):
   - Location: On the top of the foot, between the big and second toes.

- Acupressure Technique: Apply firm pressure for 2-3 minutes. This point can help with emotional balance and stress reduction.

5. Heart 7 (HT7):
   - Location: On the wrist, in line with the little finger and about one inch above the wrist crease.
   - Acupressure Technique: Gently press this point with your thumb for 2-3 minutes to reduce stress and promote relaxation.

6. Kidney 1 (KD1):
   - Location: On the sole of the foot, in the depression at the center of the sole.
   - Acupressure Technique: Apply gentle pressure with your thumb for 2-3 minutes. This point can help with emotional balance and relaxation.

When using acupressure for stress relief, focus on deep breathing, mindfulness, and maintaining a comfortable level of pressure. Remember that acupressure is not a substitute for professional treatment of depression. If you or someone you know is struggling with depression, reach out to a mental health professional for support and appropriate care. Acupressure can be a helpful complement to overall well-being but should be used in conjunction with a comprehensive treatment plan for depression.

5

Chapter 5

Conclusion

"In the journey through the world of Acupressure, we have discovered the power of touch and intention. Acupressure, an ancient healing art, has shown us that the wisdom of generations past can be harnessed to enhance our well-being in the present.

As we've explored the history, principles, and techniques of Acupressure, we've unlocked a treasure trove of knowledge that empowers us to take control of our health and vitality. The understanding of meridians, pressure points, and the flow of vital energy within our bodies has illuminated a path to self-healing and balance.

We have learned how to alleviate common ailments and discomforts, from headaches and back pain to stress and insomnia, with the gentle but powerful touch of our fingertips. We've understood that Acupressure is not just a physical practice but also a deeply holistic approach that nourishes the body, mind, and spirit.

In the quest for optimal health and harmony, we've uncovered the significance of maintaining a balanced lifestyle, embracing proper nutrition, and cultivating mindfulness. The journey of Acupressure is a journey toward self-awareness and self-care, a journey that brings us closer to our own bodies and their incredible ability to heal.

As we conclude this book on Acupressure, remember that the knowledge you've gained can be a lifelong companion, offering relief, relaxation, and restoration whenever needed. Continue to explore and practice Acupressure, share it with others, and let its benefits ripple through your life and the lives of those you touch.

May the wisdom of Acupressure guide you on a path of well-being and harmony. Your journey toward better health and a more balanced life has just begun. Embrace it with open hands, an open heart, and the knowledge that the power to heal and transform lies within you. Thank you for taking this transformative journey with us."